# Quantum Well Being Strategy

## Anti-Ageing + Weight Loss + Well-being Strategy

# It's not Just About Dieting!

**This is the Anti-Ageing Weight Loss and well being Strategy you have been waiting for all this time**

**All you have to do is to "Do it Eat it Feel it Look young live it and tell your story".**

Healthy-living is one of the key factors in your well-being.

# Why is this so important?

Because when you think about it, what is the biggest most expensive part of your life that eats away at your wellbeing the most? In most cases it is the wrong food that you eat that eats away your wellbeing and later on takes money straight out of your pocket to treat the problems caused by the wrong things you eat.

Are you looking for a strategy which will enable you to eat to stay young, feel healthy and loss weight to live it at the same time and tell your story? Then look no further!

There is a proven eating strategy which will enable you to eat yourself young. What you really need to achieve may come as a surprise to you.

Did you know that good bacteria improves the health of your digestive track and bowels and can also determine how you look too?

"Healthy bacteria make up the main components of the skin's protective mantle" (Cheda Mikic, reveals). If these levels become depleted, your skin is prone to irritation and inflammation. This increases the release of free radicals and the enzyme collagens, which breaks down skin-plumping collagen.

Both of these effects lead to long term ageing, but reduced bacteria levels will also make you look older right now, because it results in drier skin, which can make you look far older than your years".

Another startling recent discovery is that when the pro-biotic bacteria on the surface of your skin feed on the pre-biotic bacteria they live alongside, and produce water which boosts the skin's hydration.

# So, what does this mean?

This means that balancing bacteria levels is becoming the latest way in which you can put new strength to your skin.

Did you know that Skincare companies are now actually encouraging this by adding pro-biotic to their products?

You can boost your skin's health and appearance and also increase levels of good bacteria in the gut by boosting your diet levels.

Essentially, this will improve your digestion, immunity, energy and stress levels, and eventually your sleep habits.

Recent trials by the University of Reading showed that you can increase your bug levels by over 133 million in just five days by eating foods high in pre-biotic, such as bananas, oats and onions.

 "Antioxidant foods have many benefits in promoting healthy, younger-looking skin".  "Antioxidants neutralize skin-harming free radicals and they are not only effective when applied topically".

Dr Sach Mohan (anti-ageing skin clinics Renew Medica): refers to The Clinical Nutrition trial, which found that a healthy intake of a fat found in nuts and seeds was as important as vitamin C in making skin look younger, as it helps boost hydration, 'so fine lines puff up and become less noticeable'.

Recent research published in the American Journal of Clinical Nutrition, indicates that women over 40 with highest amount of vitamin C in their diet were 11% less likely to develop wrinkles than those with low levels.

# So, what do you need to do?

- Eat regular servings of pro-biotic foods: e.g. live yoghurt or Yakult.
- Eat high levels of pre-biotic foods, to help the bacteria in your system to thrive.
- Eat Antioxidant foods: - fruits and vegetables particularly the ones high in vitamin C – e.g. kiwi fruit, peppers, strawberries and citrus fruit.
- Increase the levels of healthy essential fatty acids in your diet, which are necessary for a healthy immune system and increased mental clarity.
- Drink a glass of warm water with half a lemon or lime juice to start the day.
- Drink at least 2 litres or 8 more glasses of water a day; a cup of herbal or green tea, with skimmed milk and a glass of fruit juice.

# So, what do you need to avoid?

- You need to avoid sugary drinks altogether. Dr Perricone, author of 'The Perricone Weight-loss diet' confirms that sugar actually makes your skin look older.

- You also need to avoid coffee as this can lead to elevated levels of cortisol and insulin, which locks in body fat and weight gain.

# Conclusion

To Summarize, boosting the levels of Healthy essential fatty acids in your diet is important. These are necessary for a healthy immune system. A combination of the "*So, what do you need to?*" might sound complicated, but in reality it is not. A daily intake of two to three portions of pro/pre-biotic foods, five portions of fruit and vegetables, and one or two portions of oily fish, seeds or their oils, and nuts will do it.

This anti-ageing weight loss strategy puts together valuable information which you need to help you on your to eat it, look younger and lose weight at the same time. This strategy guides you to have a daily eating pattern broken down to a Breakfast, Lunch and Dinner.

You can find most of the items of food and fruits you need in most supermarkets around you. This anti-ageing weight loss strategy publication puts together a gallery of most of the items you need.

Without further ado, you have below a seven day anti-ageing weight loss eating strategy you need to maintain your "well-being" through "Healthy-Living".

# Essentials

## Step One

To really power things up, you have to start by cleansing your Colon to get rid of all the toxins you have accumulated over the years.

Plaque is the result of years of eating chemically enhanced and treated foods. It eventually forms a solid wall coating your insides that causes significant harm and even disease.

The Royal Society of Medicine has correctly determined that **"death begins in the colon."** And this same harmful plaque is the chief cause! Therefore you MUST get rid of it before it forever gets rid of you.

Many people are reporting that once this plaque is gone, they:

**1.** Suddenly feel better

**2.** Have more energy

**3.** Lose lots of fat and weight!

**4.** And all WITHOUT dieting in the slightest.

## Step Two

Take Chocolate (Choxi+) as part of your snack. Choxi+ is high antioxidant brand which has shown to help improve skin hydration. It makes the skin to look smoother and even helps to protect it against UV damage. By swapping one of the snacks mentioned in your daily food intake for three squares of Choxi+, will be fantastic indeed.

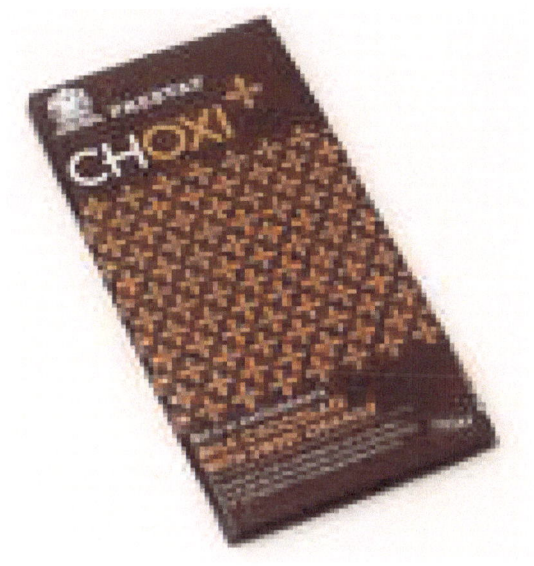

## Step Three

Take Pure Evening Primrose Oil, (Efamol) 90 x 500mg capsules daily. Evening Primrose oil is best known for its ability to help with hormonal issues such as PMS or tender breasts, but it is also a potent skin firmer. According to trials in Germany, taking six 500mg capsules of Evening Primrose Oil daily for just twelve weeks will result to 20% more moisture in the skin. It means it will look firmer, smoother and younger.

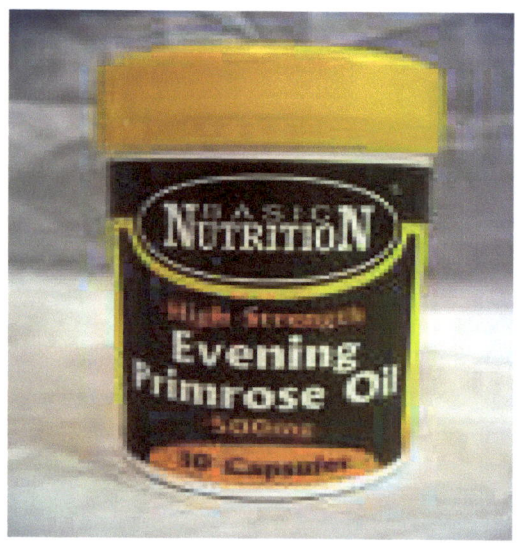

## Step Four

Take a glass of warm water with lime or lemon juice first thing each morning followed by 8 glasses of water and a glass of fruit juice during the day

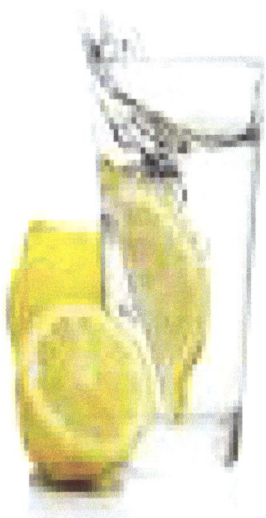

## Step Five

Follow this 7 Day Eating pattern to gain the maximum results you need.

### DAY 1

#### BREAKFAST:

- Scrambled eggs (two eggs)
- 50g of smoked salmon
- A slice of toasted wholemeal bread.
- A snack of Actimel – Style Yoghurt drink

#### LUNCH:

- Watercress Salad
- Sliced papaya
- 6 drained Marinated Artichokes
- 50g of low-fat feta
- Dress it with one table spoon balsamic vinegar and walnut or olive oil.
- Serve with 3 oatcakes.
- A Snack of one Apple

#### DINNER

- 1 red pepper filled with:
- A mixture of 50g (dry weight) couscous,
- ¼ of an onion
- ½ a courgette
- A dash of olive oil.
- Bake in the oven at 200°C/180°C fan/Gas 6 until the pepper softens.
- Serve with Peas and a dab of Mustard.
- A snack of one small handful of nuts

# Recipe – DAY 1

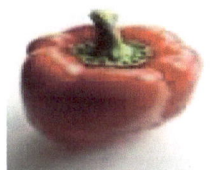
**Red Pepper**

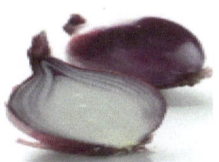
**Red Onion**

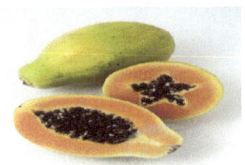
**Papaya**

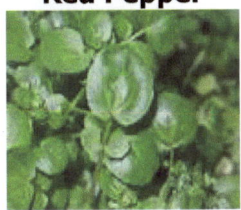
**Watercress**

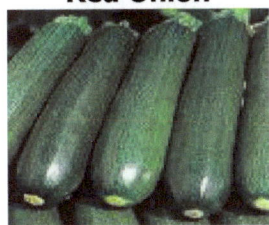
**Courgette**

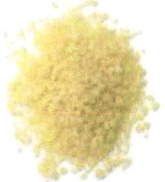
**Couscous**

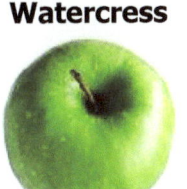
**Apple**

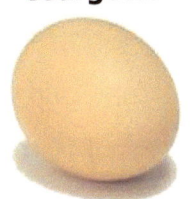
**Eggs**

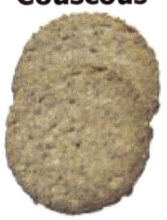
**Oatcakes**

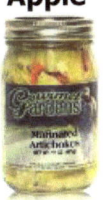
**Marinated Artichokes**

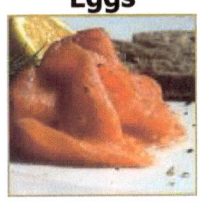
**smoked salmon**

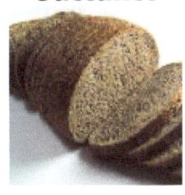
**Wholemeal bread**

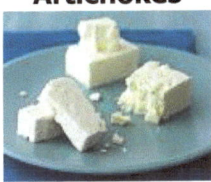
**Low-Fat Feta**

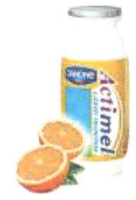
**Actimel Yoghurt drink**

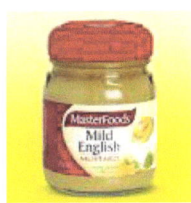
**Mustard**

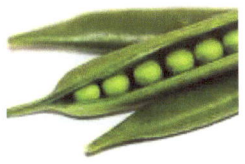
**Peas**

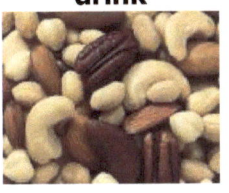
**Nuts**

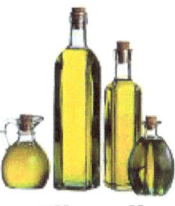
**Olive oil**

# DAY 2

## BREAKFAST:

- 40g Oates and water Porridge
- Topped with 3 handfuls of any sliced berry
- One handful of walnuts.
- A snack of Actimel – Style yoghurt drink

## LUNCH:

- 400g French Onion Can-Soup
- Two pieces of toasted wholemeal bread
- 4 Artichokes mashed
- A little low-fat yoghurt.
- A snack of 2 Oatcakes topped with low-sugar jam

## DINNER:

- 125g grilled salmon or
- Trout splashed with lemon juice and a dash of olive oil.
- Baby Spinach Salad
- Cherry Tomatoes
- Sweetcorn topped
- 4 sliced new potatoes.
- One peace of fruit

# Recipe – DAY 2

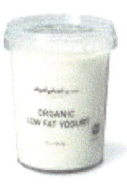

**low-fat yoghurt**

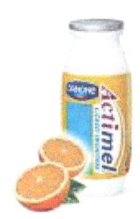

**Actimel Yoghurt drink**

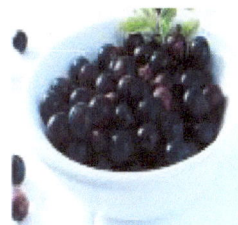

**Berry**

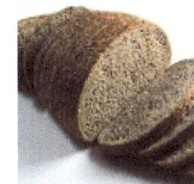

**Wholemeal bread**

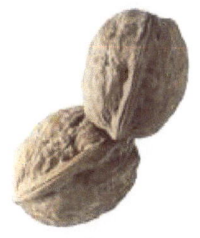

**Walnuts**

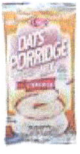

**Oates**

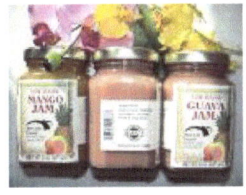

**Low Suger Jam**

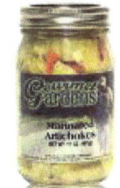

**Marinated Artichokes**

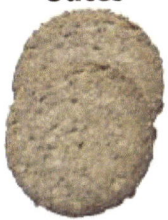

**Oatcakes**

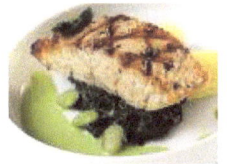

**Grilled Salmon**

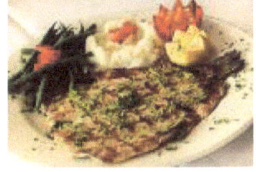

**Grilled Trout**

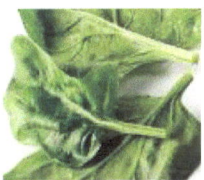

**Baby Spinach**

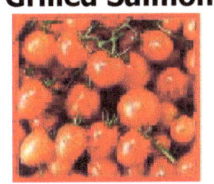

**Cherry Tomatoes**

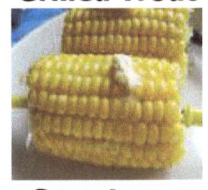

**Sweetcorn**

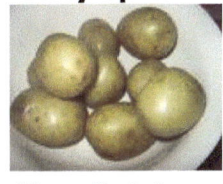

**New Potatoes**

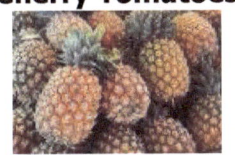

**Pineapples**

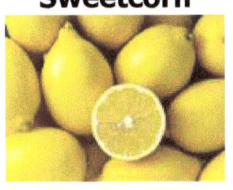

**Lemon**

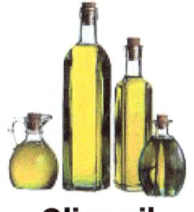

**Olive oil**

# DAY 3

## BREAKFAST:

- 150g pot Greek yoghurt mixed with:
- One teaspoon of honey
- One chopped banana
- One tablespoon of Oates.
- A snack of 2 Kiwi fruit

## LUNCH:

- 200g jacket potato with:
- Two tablespoon of low-fat coleslaw
- One tablespoon of peanuts
- A green salad.
- A snack of 125g pot of low-fat yoghurt

## DINNER:

- 100g chicken cut into small chunks.
- Fry in a little olive oil with ¼ of an onion
- Some garlic until softened.
- Add 100g canned tomatoes,
- Sliced red and yellow peppers
- 6 chopped olives
- Add some paprika spices.
- Simmer for 15 minutes.
- Serve with 50g dry weight Brown Rice.
- A snack of One Quaker Oat Bar

# Recipe – DAY 3

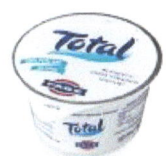

**pot Greek yoghurt**

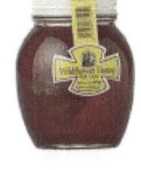

**Honey**

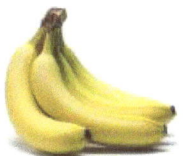

**Banana**

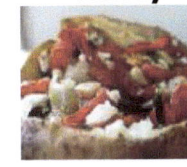

**Jacket Potato**

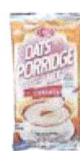

**Oates**

Kiwi Fruit

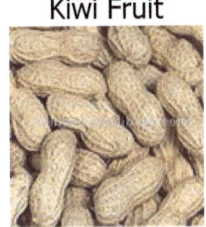

Kiwi Fruit

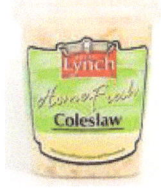

**Coleslaw**

**Pot Low-fat Yoghurt**

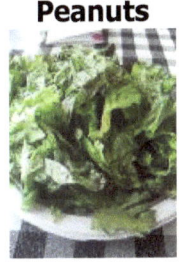

**Peanuts**

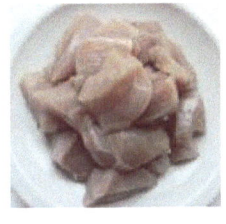

**Chicken Cut**

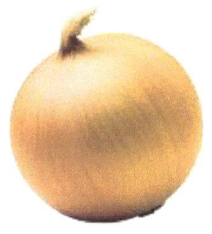

**Onion**

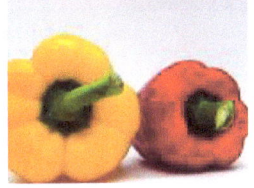

**Green Salad**

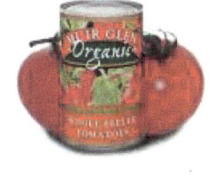

**Canned Tomatoes**

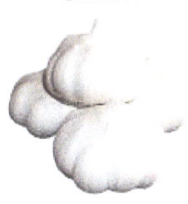

**Garlic**

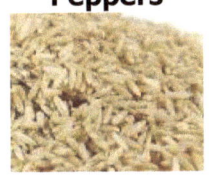

**Red & Yellow Peppers**

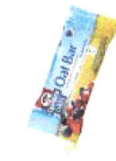

**Brown Rice**

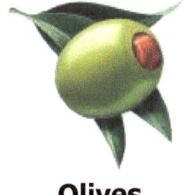

**Quaker Oat Bar**

**Olives**

# DAY 4

## BREAKFAST:

- One peach
- 2 kiwi fruit
- A handful of strawberries
- Made into a fruit salad mixed with one Actimel-style yoghurt drink
- A snack of one handful nuts.

## LUNCH:

- 150g of vegetable quiche served with:
- Salad of spinach
- Cherry tomatoes
- Red onion, topped with,
- One tablespoon of balsamic vinegar
- And a little olive oil.
- A snack of 2 Oatcakes + 1 mini Babybel cheese

## DINNER:

- 100g grilled Gammon Steak
- Serve with Swede or Cauliflower boiled then mashed with;
- Some chopped Spring Onion,
- Parsley
- A little low-fat yoghurt
- Unlimited boiled Leeks.
- A snack of one Pear or Peach

# Recipe – DAY 4

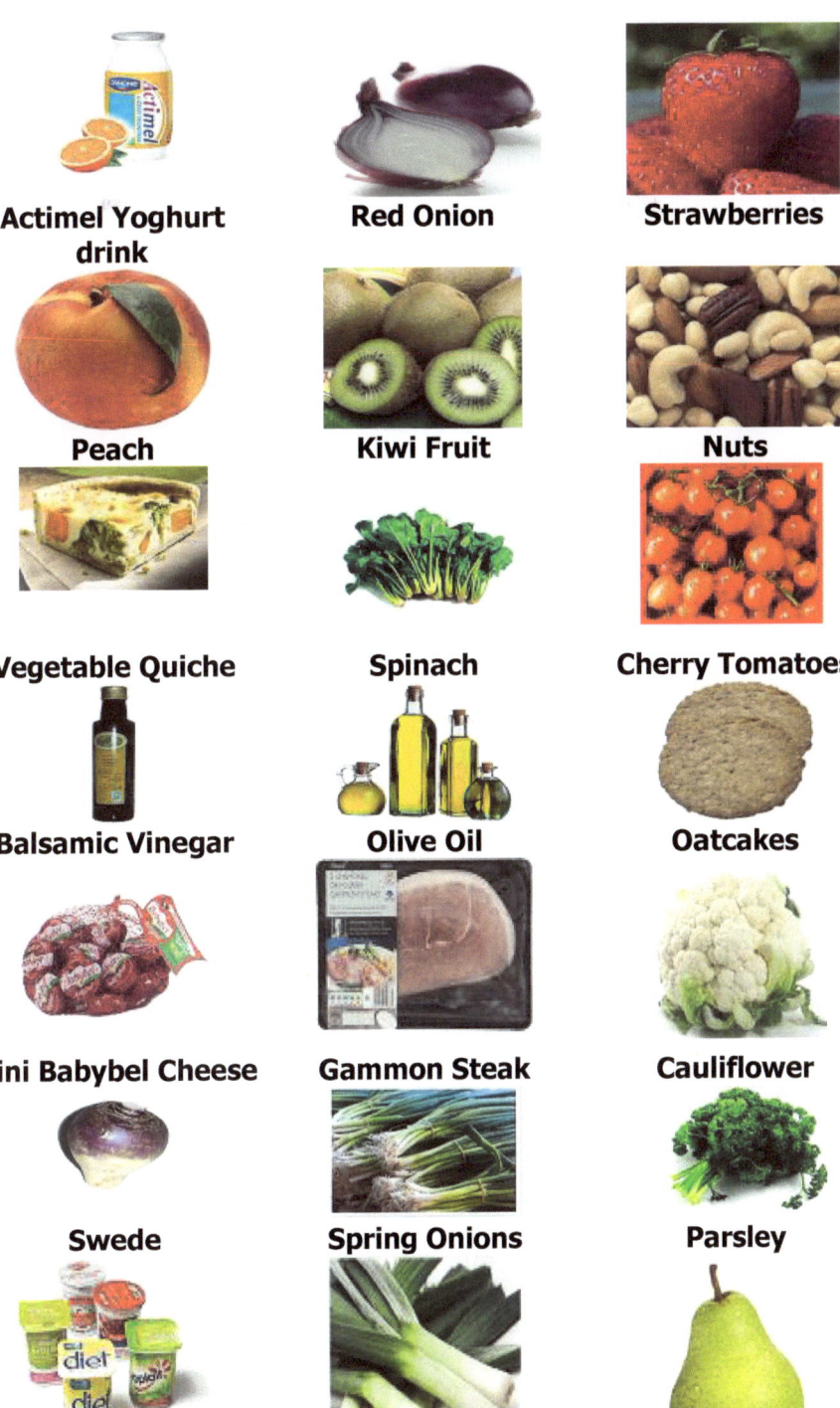

| | | |
|---|---|---|
| Actimel Yoghurt drink | Red Onion | Strawberries |
| Peach | Kiwi Fruit | Nuts |
| Vegetable Quiche | Spinach | Cherry Tomatoes |
| Balsamic Vinegar | Olive Oil | Oatcakes |
| Mini Babybel Cheese | Gammon Steak | Cauliflower |
| Swede | Spring Onions | Parsley |
| Low-fat Yoghurt | Leeks | Pear |

# DAY 5

## BREAKFAST:

- 2 pieces of toasted wholemeal bread topped with,
- 1 mashed banana.
- 125g pot low-fat natural yoghurt.
- A snack of 2 Kiwi fruit

## LUNCH:

- Toss a selection of red pepper,
- Onion
- Aubergine
- One tablespoon Olive Oil,
- Then roast in the oven or grill until they soften and slightly char.
- Stuff into a small Wholemeal Pitta bread with:
- One tablespoon low-fat Houmous
- Serve with a small Chinese leaves Salad.
- A snack of one Actimel –Style yoghurt drink.

## DINNER:

- Kebab of 100g Grilled firm white fish
- Served with Cherry Tomatoes
- Marinated artichokes,
- Onion.
- Serve with one tablespoon Tzatziki
- 50g of dry weight couscous.
- A snack of one handful of Nuts

# Recipe – DAY 5

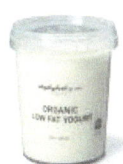

**low-fat yoghurt**

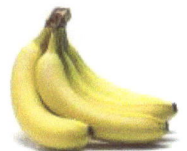

**Banana**

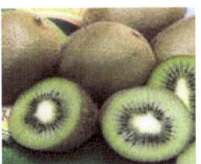

**Kiwi Fruit**

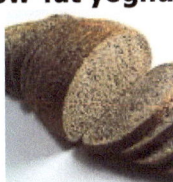

**Wholemeal bread**

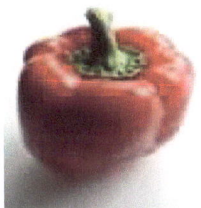

**Red Pepper**

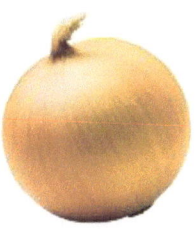

**Onion**

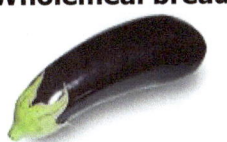

**Aubergine**

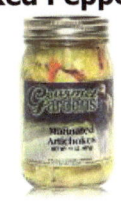

**Marinated Artichokes**

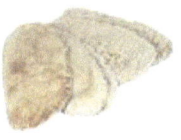

**Pitta Bread**

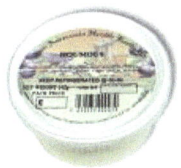

**Low-fat Houmous**

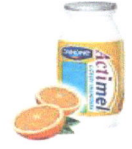

**Actimel Yoghurt drink**

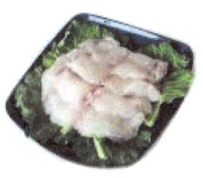

**Firm White Fish**

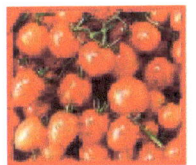

**Cherry Tomatoes**

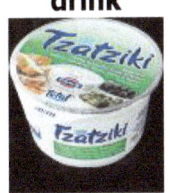

**Tzatziki**

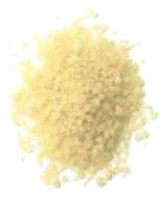

**Couscous**

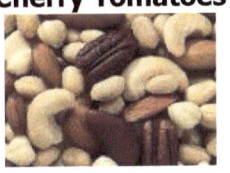

**Nuts**

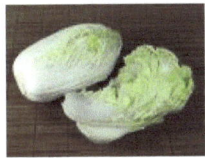

**Chinese Leaves Salad**

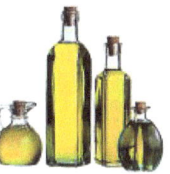

**Olive oil**

# DAY 6

## BREAKFAST:

- Two Weetabix Cereal
- Served with 150ml Skimmed Milk
- 3 Handfuls of Berries.
- A snack of 125g tub of Low-Fat Yoghurt

## LUNCH:

- Frittata
- Made with 2 eggs,
- A handful of Butter Beans
- Spinach
- And chopped Red Pepper.
- Mix the ingredients together and cook in a frying pan
- On a low heat until it firms through
- Grill the top to finish.
- Serve with 200g Low-sugar Can of baked Beans.
- Snack of 3 handfuls of any Berry.

## DINNER:

- Grilled or pan fried 100g Lean Steak
- Served with roasted Courgette
- Yellow Pepper,
- Cherry Tomato
- Onion and topped with One tablespoon Pesto.
- A snack of one Apple dipped into One teaspoon Nut Butter

# Recipe – DAY 6

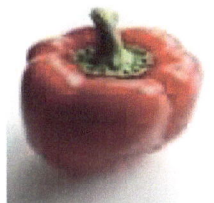

**Red Pepper**

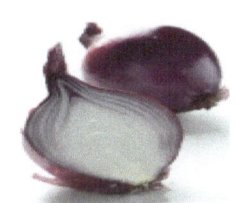

**Red Onion**

**Skimmed Milk**

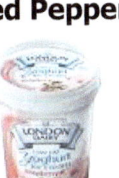

**Low-fat Yoghurt**

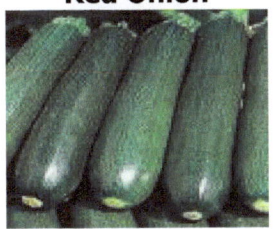

**Courgette**

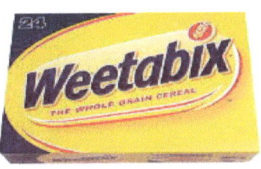

**Weetabix**

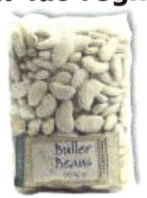

**Butter Beans**

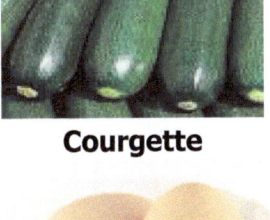

**Eggs**

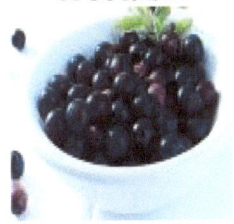

**Berry**

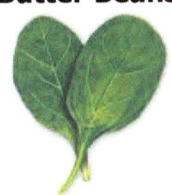

**Spinach**

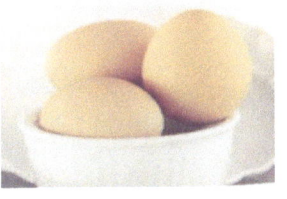

**Baked Beans**

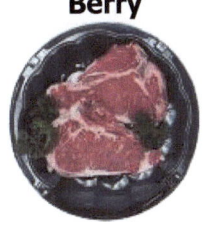

**Lean Steak**

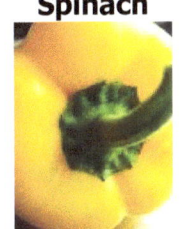

**Yellow Pepper**

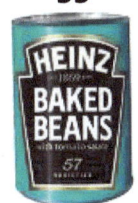

**Cherry Tomatoes**

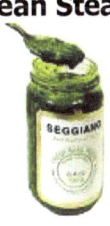

**Pesto**

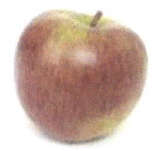

**Apple**

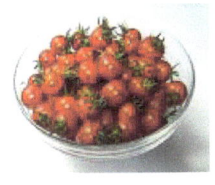

**Nut Butter**

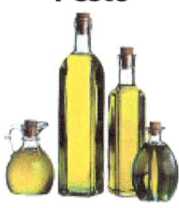

**Olive oil**

# DAY 7

## BREAKFAST:

- Two slices of wholemeal bread soaked
- In a mix of 1 egg and skimmed milk.
- Fried in a little oil spray.
- Serve with 2 handfuls of Berries or grilled Tomatoes.
- A snack of one Actimel-Style yoghurt drink

## LUNCH:

- 100g Roast Beef, pork or lamb
- Served with 2 Roast Potatoes
- Carrots,
- Cabbage
- Leeks topped with a little gravy.
- A snack of one Quaker Oat Bar

## DINNER:

- Watercress Salad
- Pear
- Strawberries with
- 50g Low-Fat Brie,
- Served with 2 Oatcakes.
- A snack of 3 handfuls of Berries

# Recipe – DAY 7

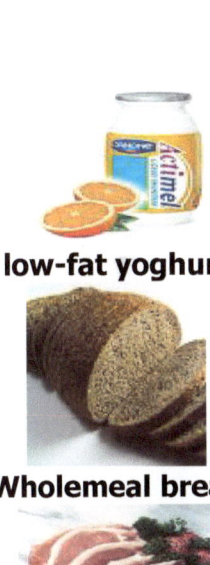
**low-fat yoghurt**

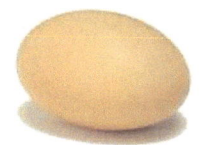
**Eggs**

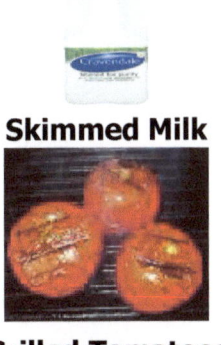
**Skimmed Milk**

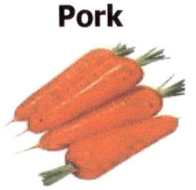
**Wholemeal bread**

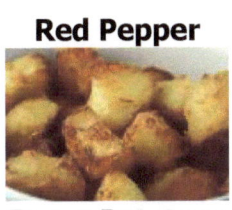
**Red Pepper**

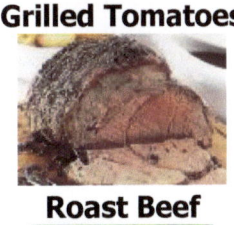
**Grilled Tomatoes**

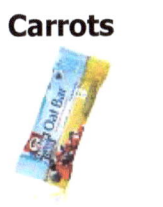
**Pork**

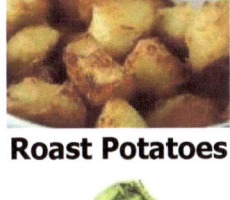
**Roast Potatoes**

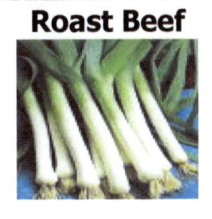
**Roast Beef**

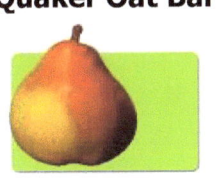
**Carrots**

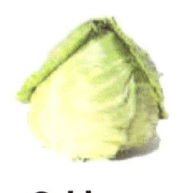
**Cabbage**

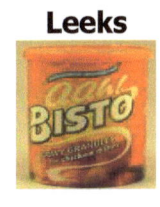
**Leeks**

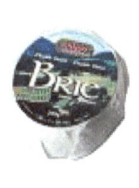
**Quaker Oat Bar**

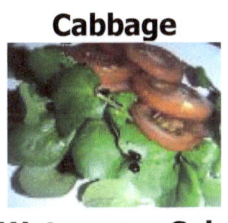
**Watercress Sala**

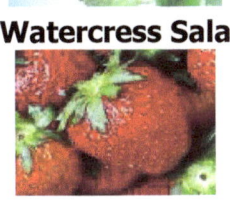
**Gravy**

**Pear**

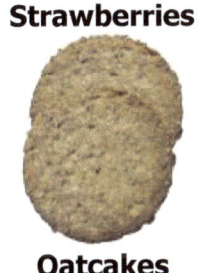
**Strawberries**

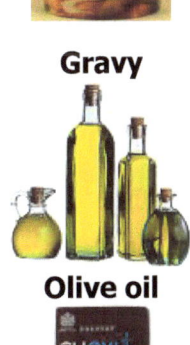
**Olive oil**

**Low-fat Brie**

**Oatcakes**

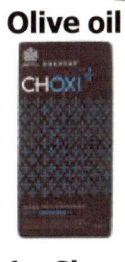
**Choxi+ Chocolate**

**Here we go!**

**You have it!**

**Eat it Feel it Look young live it and tell your story!**

www.ingramcontent.com/pod-product-compliance
Lightning Source LLC
Chambersburg PA
CBHW050927290526
45792CB00002B/909